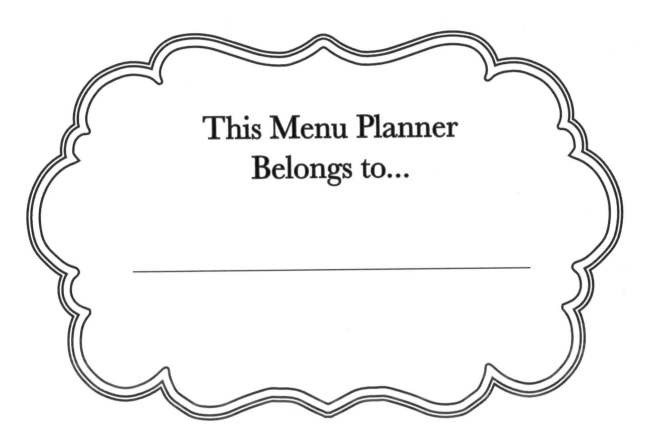

This Menu Planner
Belongs to...

_____

Meal Planner

Week of _____

	Breakfast	Lunch	Dinner	Snacks
Monday				
Tuesday				
Wednesday				
Thursday				
Friday				

	Breakfast	Lunch	Dinner	Snacks
Saturday				
Sunday				

Shopping List

Notes

Meal Planner

Week of _____

	Breakfast	Lunch	Dinner	Snacks
Monday				
Tuesday				
Wednesday				
Thursday				
Friday				

	Breakfast	Lunch	Dinner	Snacks
Saturday				
Sunday				

Shopping List

Notes

Meal Planner

Week of _____

	Breakfast	Lunch	Dinner	Snacks
Monday				
Tuesday				
Wednesday				
Thursday				
Friday				

	Breakfast	Lunch	Dinner	Snacks
Saturday				
Sunday				

Shopping List

Notes

Meal Planner

Week of _____

	Breakfast	Lunch	Dinner	Snacks
Monday				
Tuesday				
Wednesday				
Thursday				
Friday				

	Breakfast	Lunch	Dinner	Snacks
Saturday				
Sunday				

Shopping List

Notes

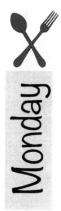

Meal Planner

Week of _____

	Breakfast	Lunch	Dinner	Snacks
Monday				
Tuesday				
Wednesday				
Thursday				
Friday				

	Breakfast	Lunch	Dinner	Snacks
Saturday				
Sunday				

Shopping List

Notes

Meal Planner

	Breakfast	Lunch	Dinner	Snacks
Monday				
Tuesday				
Wednesday				
Thursday				
Friday				

	Breakfast	Lunch	Dinner	Snacks
Saturday				
Sunday				

Shopping List

Notes

Meal Planner

Week of _____

	Breakfast	Lunch	Dinner	Snacks
Monday				
Tuesday				
Wednesday				
Thursday				
Friday				

	Breakfast	Lunch	Dinner	Snacks
Saturday				
Sunday				

Shopping List

Notes

Meal Planner

Week of _____

	Breakfast	Lunch	Dinner	Snacks
Monday				
Tuesday				
Wednesday				
Thursday				
Friday				

	Breakfast	Lunch	Dinner	Snacks
Saturday				
Sunday				

Shopping List

Notes

Meal Planner

Week of _____

	Breakfast	Lunch	Dinner	Snacks
Monday				
Tuesday				
Wednesday				
Thursday				
Friday				

	Breakfast	Lunch	Dinner	Snacks
Saturday				
Sunday				

Shopping List

Notes

Meal Planner

Week of _____

	Breakfast	Lunch	Dinner	Snacks
Monday				
Tuesday				
Wednesday				
Thursday				
Friday				

	Breakfast	Lunch	Dinner	Snacks
Saturday				
Sunday				

Shopping List

Notes

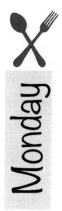

Meal Planner

Week of _____

	Breakfast	Lunch	Dinner	Snacks
Monday				
Tuesday				
Wednesday				
Thursday				
Friday				

	Breakfast	Lunch	Dinner	Snacks
Saturday				
Sunday				

Shopping List

Notes

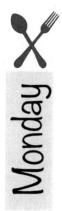

Meal Planner

Week of _____

	Breakfast	Lunch	Dinner	Snacks
Monday				
Tuesday				
Wednesday				
Thursday				
Friday				

	Breakfast	Lunch	Dinner	Snacks
Saturday				
Sunday				

Shopping List

Notes

Meal Planner

Week of _____

	Breakfast	Lunch	Dinner	Snacks
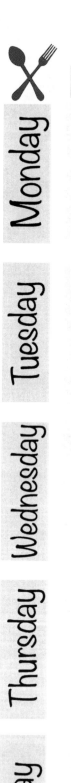Monday				
Tuesday				
Wednesday				
Thursday				
Friday				

	Breakfast	Lunch	Dinner	Snacks
Saturday				
Sunday				

Shopping List

Notes

Meal Planner

Week of _____

	Breakfast	Lunch	Dinner	Snacks
Monday				
Tuesday				
Wednesday				
Thursday				
Friday				

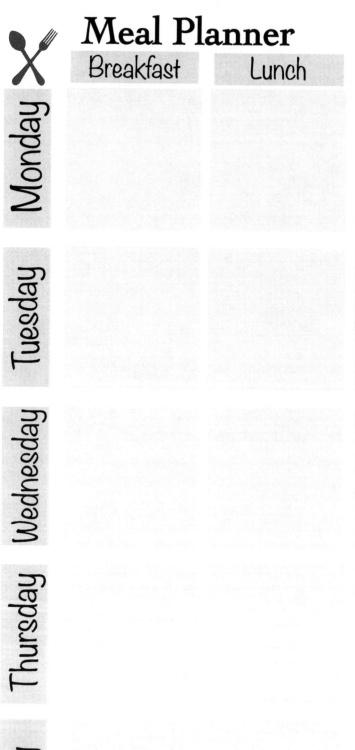

	Breakfast	Lunch	Dinner	Snacks
Saturday				
Sunday				

Shopping List

Notes

Meal Planner

Week of _____

	Breakfast	Lunch	Dinner	Snacks
Monday				
Tuesday				
Wednesday				
Thursday				
Friday				

	Breakfast	Lunch	Dinner	Snacks
Saturday				
Sunday				

Shopping List

Notes

Meal Planner

Week of _____

	Breakfast	Lunch	Dinner	Snacks
Monday				
Tuesday				
Wednesday				
Thursday				
Friday				

	Breakfast	Lunch	Dinner	Snacks
Saturday				
Sunday				

Shopping List

Notes

Meal Planner

Week of

	Breakfast	Lunch	Dinner	Snacks
Monday				
Tuesday				
Wednesday				
Thursday				
Friday				

	Breakfast	Lunch	Dinner	Snacks
Saturday				
Sunday				

Shopping List

Notes

Meal Planner

Week of _____

	Breakfast	Lunch	Dinner	Snacks
Monday				
Tuesday				
Wednesday				
Thursday				
Friday				

	Breakfast	Lunch	Dinner	Snacks
Saturday				
Sunday				

Shopping List

Notes

Meal Planner

Week of _____

	Breakfast	Lunch	Dinner	Snacks
Monday				
Tuesday				
Wednesday				
Thursday				
Friday				

	Breakfast	Lunch	Dinner	Snacks
Saturday				
Sunday				

Shopping List

Notes

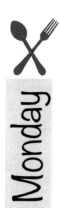

Meal Planner

Week of _____

	Breakfast	Lunch	Dinner	Snacks
Monday				
Tuesday				
Wednesday				
Thursday				
Friday				

	Breakfast	Lunch	Dinner	Snacks
Saturday				
Sunday				

Shopping List

Notes

Meal Planner

Week of _____

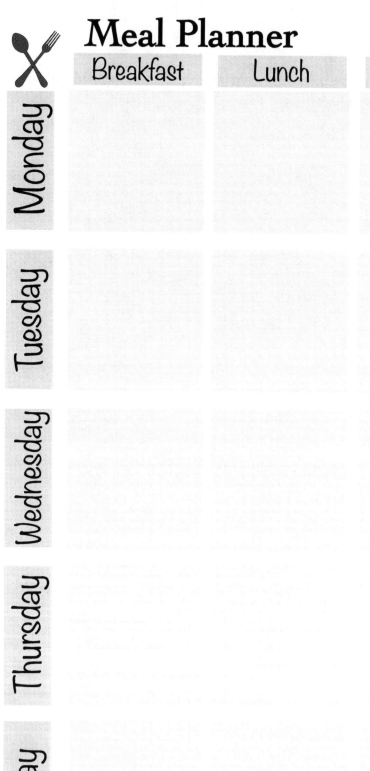

	Breakfast	Lunch	Dinner	Snacks
Monday				
Tuesday				
Wednesday				
Thursday				
Friday				

	Breakfast	Lunch	Dinner	Snacks
Saturday				
Sunday				

Shopping List

Notes

Meal Planner

Week of _____

	Breakfast	Lunch	Dinner	Snacks
Monday				
Tuesday				
Wednesday				
Thursday				
Friday				

	Breakfast	Lunch	Dinner	Snacks
Saturday				
Sunday				

Shopping List

Notes

Meal Planner

Week of _____

	Breakfast	Lunch	Dinner	Snacks
Monday				
Tuesday				
Wednesday				
Thursday				
Friday				

	Breakfast	Lunch	Dinner	Snacks
Saturday				
Sunday				

Shopping List

Notes

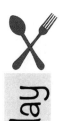

Meal Planner

Week of _____

	Breakfast	Lunch	Dinner	Snacks
Monday				
Tuesday				
Wednesday				
Thursday				
Friday				

	Breakfast	Lunch	Dinner	Snacks
Saturday				
Sunday				

Shopping List

Notes

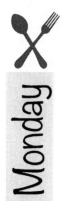

Meal Planner

Week of _____

	Breakfast	Lunch	Dinner	Snacks
Monday				
Tuesday				
Wednesday				
Thursday				
Friday				

	Breakfast	Lunch	Dinner	Snacks
Saturday				
Sunday				

Shopping List

Notes

Meal Planner

Week of _____

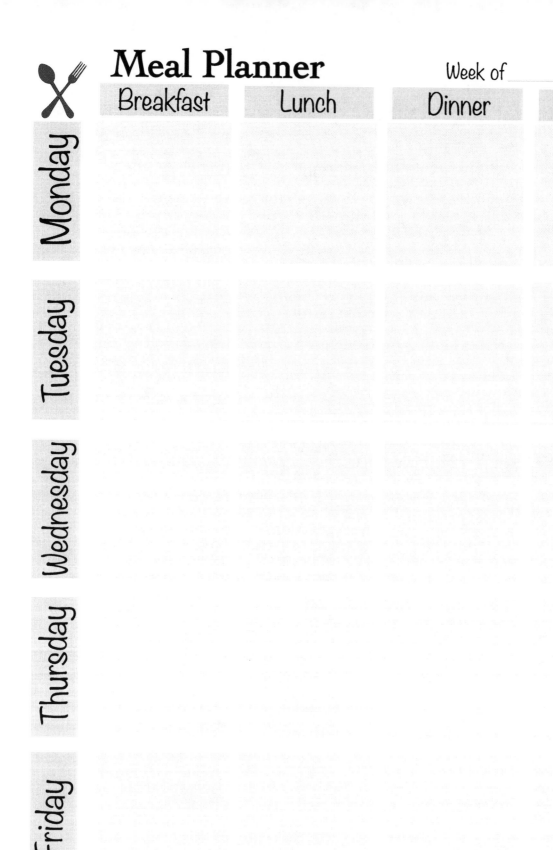

	Breakfast	Lunch	Dinner	Snacks
Monday				
Tuesday				
Wednesday				
Thursday				
Friday				

	Breakfast	Lunch	Dinner	Snacks
Saturday				
Sunday				

Shopping List

Notes

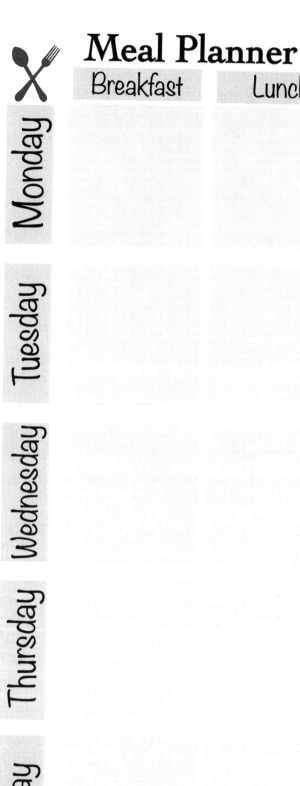

Meal Planner

Week of _____

	Breakfast	Lunch	Dinner	Snacks
Monday				
Tuesday				
Wednesday				
Thursday				
Friday				

	Breakfast	Lunch	Dinner	Snacks
Saturday				
Sunday				

Shopping List

Notes

Meal Planner

Week of _____

	Breakfast	Lunch	Dinner	Snacks
Monday				
Tuesday				
Wednesday				
Thursday				
Friday				

	Breakfast	Lunch	Dinner	Snacks
Saturday				
Sunday				

Shopping List

Notes

Meal Planner

Week of _____

	Breakfast	Lunch	Dinner	Snacks
Monday				
Tuesday				
Wednesday				
Thursday				
Friday				

	Breakfast	Lunch	Dinner	Snacks
Saturday				
Sunday				

Shopping List

Notes

Meal Planner

Week of _____

	Breakfast	Lunch	Dinner	Snacks
Monday				
Tuesday				
Wednesday				
Thursday				
Friday				

	Breakfast	Lunch	Dinner	Snacks
Saturday				
Sunday				

Shopping List

Notes

Meal Planner

Week of _____

	Breakfast	Lunch	Dinner	Snacks
Monday				
Tuesday				
Wednesday				
Thursday				
Friday				

	Breakfast	Lunch	Dinner	Snacks
Saturday				
Sunday				

Shopping List

Notes

Meal Planner

Week of _____

	Breakfast	Lunch	Dinner	Snacks
Monday				
Tuesday				
Wednesday				
Thursday				
Friday				

	Breakfast	Lunch	Dinner	Snacks
Saturday				
Sunday				

Shopping List

Notes

Meal Planner

Week of _____

	Breakfast	Lunch	Dinner	Snacks
Monday				
Tuesday				
Wednesday				
Thursday				
Friday				

	Breakfast	Lunch	Dinner	Snacks
Saturday				
Sunday				

Shopping List

Notes

Meal Planner

Week of _____

	Breakfast	Lunch	Dinner	Snacks
Monday				
Tuesday				
Wednesday				
Thursday				
Friday				

	Breakfast	Lunch	Dinner	Snacks
Saturday				
Sunday				

Shopping List

Notes

Meal Planner

Week of _____

	Breakfast	Lunch	Dinner	Snacks
Monday				
Tuesday				
Wednesday				
Thursday				
Friday				

	Breakfast	Lunch	Dinner	Snacks
Saturday				
Sunday				

Shopping List

Notes

Meal Planner

Week of _____

	Breakfast	Lunch	Dinner	Snacks
Monday				
Tuesday				
Wednesday				
Thursday				
Friday				

	Breakfast	Lunch	Dinner	Snacks
Saturday				
Sunday				

Shopping List

Notes

Meal Planner

Week of _____

	Breakfast	Lunch	Dinner	Snacks
Monday				
Tuesday				
Wednesday				
Thursday				
Friday				

	Breakfast	Lunch	Dinner	Snacks
Saturday				
Sunday				

Shopping List

Notes

Meal Planner

Week of _____

	Breakfast	Lunch	Dinner	Snacks
Monday				
Tuesday				
Wednesday				
Thursday				
Friday				

	Breakfast	Lunch	Dinner	Snacks
Saturday				
Sunday				

Shopping List

Notes

Meal Planner

Week of _____

	Breakfast	Lunch	Dinner	Snacks
Monday				
Tuesday				
Wednesday				
Thursday				
Friday				

	Breakfast	Lunch	Dinner	Snacks
Saturday				
Sunday				

Shopping List

Notes

Meal Planner

Week of _____

	Breakfast	Lunch	Dinner	Snacks
Monday				
Tuesday				
Wednesday				
Thursday				
Friday				

	Breakfast	Lunch	Dinner	Snacks
Saturday				
Sunday				

Shopping List

Notes

Meal Planner

Week of _____

	Breakfast	Lunch	Dinner	Snacks
Monday				
Tuesday				
Wednesday				
Thursday				
Friday				

	Breakfast	Lunch	Dinner	Snacks
Saturday				
Sunday				

Shopping List

Notes

Meal Planner

Week of _____

	Breakfast	Lunch	Dinner	Snacks
Monday				
Tuesday				
Wednesday				
Thursday				
Friday				

	Breakfast	Lunch	Dinner	Snacks
Saturday				
Sunday				

Shopping List

Notes

Meal Planner

Week of _____

	Breakfast	Lunch	Dinner	Snacks
Monday				
Tuesday				
Wednesday				
Thursday				
Friday				

	Breakfast	Lunch	Dinner	Snacks
Saturday				
Sunday				

Shopping List

Notes

Meal Planner

Week of _____

	Breakfast	Lunch	Dinner	Snacks
Monday				
Tuesday				
Wednesday				
Thursday				
Friday				

	Breakfast	Lunch	Dinner	Snacks
Saturday				
Sunday				

Shopping List

Notes

Meal Planner

Week of _____

	Breakfast	Lunch	Dinner	Snacks
Monday				
Tuesday				
Wednesday				
Thursday				
Friday				

	Breakfast	Lunch	Dinner	Snacks
Saturday				
Sunday				

Shopping List

Notes

Meal Planner

Week of _____

	Breakfast	Lunch	Dinner	Snacks
Monday				
Tuesday				
Wednesday				
Thursday				
Friday				

	Breakfast	Lunch	Dinner	Snacks
Saturday				
Sunday				

Shopping List

Notes

Meal Planner

Week of _____

	Breakfast	Lunch	Dinner	Snacks
Monday				
Tuesday				
Wednesday				
Thursday				
Friday				

	Breakfast	Lunch	Dinner	Snacks
Saturday				
Sunday				

Shopping List

Notes

Meal Planner

Week of _____

	Breakfast	Lunch	Dinner	Snacks
Monday				
Tuesday				
Wednesday				
Thursday				
Friday				

	Breakfast	Lunch	Dinner	Snacks
Saturday				
Sunday				

Shopping List

Notes

Meal Planner

Week of _____

	Breakfast	Lunch	Dinner	Snacks
Monday				
Tuesday				
Wednesday				
Thursday				
Friday				

	Breakfast	Lunch	Dinner	Snacks
Saturday				
Sunday				

Shopping List

Notes

Meal Planner

Week of _____

	Breakfast	Lunch	Dinner	Snacks
Monday				
Tuesday				
Wednesday				
Thursday				
Friday				

	Breakfast	Lunch	Dinner	Snacks
Saturday				
Sunday				

Shopping List

Notes

Meal Planner

Week of _____

	Breakfast	Lunch	Dinner	Snacks
Monday				
Tuesday				
Wednesday				
Thursday				
Friday				

	Breakfast	Lunch	Dinner	Snacks
Saturday				
Sunday				

Shopping List

Notes

Meal Planner

Week of _____

	Breakfast	Lunch	Dinner	Snacks
Monday				
Tuesday				
Wednesday				
Thursday				
Friday				

	Breakfast	Lunch	Dinner	Snacks
Saturday				
Sunday				

Shopping List

Notes

Made in the USA
Middletown, DE
10 October 2023

40560695R00060